Ken & Eileen

If You Wear Out Your Body,
Where Will You Live?

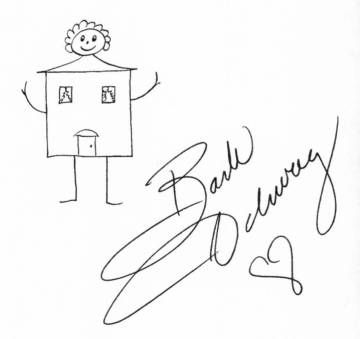

If You Wear Out Your Body, Where Will You Live?

The Little Book of Nourishment
for
Your Body, Mind, and Soul

Barb Schwarz, CSP

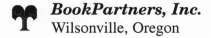

BookPartners, Inc.
Wilsonville, Oregon

Disclosure

The information in this book is for educational purposes only and is offered only as information for use in maintaining and promoting optimum health. It is not presented with the intention of diagnosing or prescribing.

For any serious health conditions the reader is advised to seek medical attention from a qualified health practitioner, such as a doctor. The author and the publisher assume no responsibility for the choices readers make pertaining to their own health conditions and/or treatment.

BookPartners, Inc.
P.O. Box 922
Wilsonville, Oregon 97070

To Andrea, my daughter.
Your innocence, your trust, your love,
and your persistence
inspires me every day.
You are my greatest teacher.

I Love You

To affect the quality of the day, that is the art of life.

— Henry David Thoreau

Acknowledgments and ...
"I Love You"

To my husband and partner Kirk Bohrer, I love you and thank you for being there with me no matter where we traveled and worked. Your undying love, understanding ways, and devotion have been the anchor and the joy of my life. You are my hero, and you light up my life!

To my dear loving friends and family, thank you for your steadfast love and support. You know who you are because you have encouraged and inspired me in my life's journey. I feel your love and you are the angels in my life.

To you all ... thank you for enriching my life and for helping me grow.

I love you,

Barb

What is now proved was once only imagined.

– William Blake

Table of Contents

Life is either a daring adventure or nothing.

– Helen Keller

Introduction

~ ~ ~ ~ ~ ~ ~ ~ ~ ~ ~ ~ ~ ~

As the reader, you have the right to know what qualifies me to write about integrating mind, body and spirit to improve personal excellence. My answer is a subjective one, which always is the case about personal discoveries.

I lived for more than forty years before I was able to put my thoughts together to form an action plan that would permit me to become closer to the kind of woman I could admire and project to others. I was able to accomplish this improvement only after I spent countless hours reading about how we think and believe affects our bodies. It is absolutely true! How you think

~ ~

and what you believe about your biological, mental and spiritual self will determine the health of your mind, body and spirit. I'm living proof that if a person opens her mind, heart and soul to the power of the Universe, that person will become a reflection of that power.

Since we humans are reluctant to accept change in another person without proof, I'd like you to turn to page 82 of this little book and look at two photographs of me. The first one is the "old" me, the person I was before I learned about nutrition for the body and nourishment for the mind and soul. When I became the "new" me I was forty pounds lighter; I'm told I look twenty years younger, and I have become happier, more in tune with the image of me as projected by the power of the Universe.

Even without the change of hair color, don't you see a remarkable difference in the youth and vibrancy of the "new" me compared to the "old" me?

So what I'm asking you to accept is that change, personal improvement, grand personal excellence in mind, body and spirit can be yours if you choose to follow the road I, and many others, have discovered. I want to share my personal discoveries with you. I want to be the pathfinder who takes your hand and leads you

~ ~

along the path to self-discovery. It is an adventure from which, once you start, there is no turning back. You will never be the same person who started on the road to expanded awareness, even if you falter and stop along the way.

My goal in writing this book is to make it easy for you to nourish your body, mind and soul on a daily basis. Many things have been written about these three parts of your makeup, as if each exists independent of the other. The fact is, body, mind and spirit are integrated aspects of the whole self, and if you seek ultimate good health, you must learn to respect who you are and take care of yourself. That's what this little book is about. If you follow the principles you learn here, you will live longer, healthier, and more joyously.

As you read this book, stay open. A closed mind is like a parachute. It doesn't work if it doesn't open. Should you come to a principle or idea that concerns you, stay with it. That tells you there is something underlying the idea or principle that you need to work on. Just read and let the understandings that are bound to follow evolve.

I love what Norman Cousins wrote about reading a book. It is a joint effort — the author's and the reader's:

~ ~

The way a book is read — which is to say, the qualities a reader brings to a book — can have as much to do with its worth as anything the author puts into it.

I urge you to read this little book with an open mind and the willingness to discover how to nourish your body, mind and spirit in a manner that will add zest, sparkle and new energy to your whole being.

That's what happened to me when I found out how to integrate my body, mind and soul in a unified effort of health, wholeness and spiritual uplift.

1

What Are You Waiting For?
This is Not a Dress Rehearsal!

~ ~ ~ ~ ~ ~ ~ ~ ~ ~ ~ ~ ~ ~

When I think of developing wholeness in life I think of three nourishing goals:
- Building your body nutritionally to perform as you were created.
- Empowering your mind to create the life you want.
- Awakening your spirit to experience a truly joyous life.

All three of these goals represent the purpose of this book. And, together with your permission, we will investigate how to maximize your bodily health, open your mind to new ideas that will give you more personal

~ ~

power, and explore the path that will lead to the expansion of your spirit.

Before we start with information on how to improve the nutrition of your body, I'd like to share a poem I keep on my refrigerator. I refer to it often, and it always reminds me that "my life is not a dress rehearsal." I do not know who wrote it, but when I read it, it always reminds me of what my true perspective should be every day.

This Day is Mine

This is the day that belongs to me, for it was given
to me early in the morning, freely and without
obligation. The moment that I accepted the gift,
I accepted the responsibility for its growth.

I received it in good condition, fresh and
young and clean,
and now that it is mine, I can choose what kind
of day it will become. I can make it ugly
by deciding to be miserable, or I can
make it beautiful by deciding to be glad.

This is the day to be happy. I know I can be just as
contented as I wish to be. Above all, I can find
contentment now, instead of thinking it is necessary
to wait for some uncertain, future pleasure.

This day is to be free, to cut the bonds of all those
tomorrows and all those yesterdays. I would be
unwise to waste any part of today in useless guilt
or distress about yesterday, or in pointless
worry or panic about tomorrow.

This is the day to treat life as
a great adventure and each moment of it as a
satisfying, rewarding experience. Since I have but
one chance at today, I want to live it fully, and
I want to live it well. I hope that I will
handle myself in such a manner that when today
becomes yesterday, my memories will be pleasant, and
when tomorrow becomes today, my regrets will be few.

On this day, I do not want to indulge in crippling
selfish emotions such as anger, hatred, and fear;
I want instead to seek their opposites.

~ ~

This is the day to be thankful, for some
pains removed and some blessings received;
to translate my gratitude from mere words into
cheerful, whole-hearted achievement.

This is the day to promise myself that I am going
to build my world with gladness and with love —
right now — because this is the only day
that belongs to me.

— Author unknown

Your Body

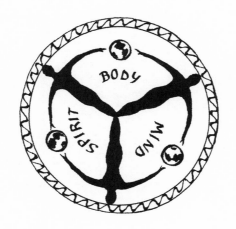

2

Rebuilding it Right!

~ ~ ~ ~ ~ ~ ~ ~ ~ ~ ~ ~ ~ ~

A moment's insight is sometimes worth a life's experience.

— Oliver Wendell Holmes

I hired a nutritionist a number of years ago when I decided to improve the condition of my body's wellness. I wanted to rebuild it right. I had suffered for years from allergies, sinus infections, ear infections, yo-yo dieting, asthma, chronic constipation, and too many colds and bouts with the flu. Does this sound familiar to you? I thought so. If my own particular health problems don't ring a bell, I know you've got your own set of

~ ~

health challenges. The concepts and ideas I learned from the nutritionist, plus the work and studying I have done on my own since then, have changed my life. I call these concepts "Recipes for Body Wellness."

They work. I am now symptom free. I don't get the colds or flus of the season, and I am in contact with thousands of people each year as I speak across the country. Because of what I learned from the nutritionist and from my own investigation, which I share with you in this book, I no longer get constipated, no longer do I get allergies or sinus infections, and the asthma that plagued me is gone. I have lost forty pounds, and I have kept it off. That is a big deal to me. What you are about to read and learn can change your life also. It certainly has changed me. Remember: Your body is the house where your spirit lives.

Since your body is the temple that houses your mind and soul, I am going to reflect on it here and on the description my nutritionist gave me about "sludge buildup" in the body and how an "intestinal cleanse" is an important way to start improving the body.

She gave me two impressive medical facts:

1. Approximately 90 percent of all diseases start in the colon.

~ ~

2. More than sixty degenerative diseases can be traced to the colon.

Having given me this information, she went on to make another point about the fact that the human body operates normally at 98.6 degrees Fahrenheit. At this temperature, a steak left on the kitchen counter would rot! All of us have a disposal plant on the inside, and when it is not moving properly, the distribution center — the colon — is clogged. Waste backs up, and this causes self-poisoning. When the colon walls become encrusted, intoxication happens with uneliminated fecal matter, and the body cannot absorb the vital nutrients it needs from the food it consumes. Unhealthy bacteria thrives in the colon when this takes place, and the body begins to absorb the toxins into the bloodstream through blood capillaries lining the colon. Then the cells, organs and tissues are exposed to these poisons. The overall body performance is lowered, and the stage is set for illness.

Yes, the colon is important; it is the key to your health. I've come to believe that your health begins and ends in the colon. In fact, the second killer of men in America today is colon cancer.

This next question is important: How many meals does the average American eat each day? Most of us

~ ~

were raised to consume three meals: breakfast, lunch, and dinner. And, of course, the refuse from these meals must be eliminated. Not the kind of subject that is popular at the average cocktail party, but we need to discuss it now. This brings us to the question: How many bowel movements does the average American have a day?

For most people, it is one. Now wait a minute. You consume three meals a day and have one bowel movement. If you put three trains on three tracks and they went into a tunnel and only one train came out, you would have two trains stuck in the tunnel. I hope you get the point!

Your intestinal tract is approximately twenty-eight feet long, including the colon. That is a lot of feet stuffed on the inside of you. Did you know that research has proved that when you eat a big, juicy piece of meat, small parts of it can be traced in your intestines for as long as seven years? There are a lot of corners, twists and turns in all those feet of intestine. What is the temperature on the inside of the colon?

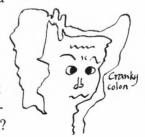

~ ~

Warm enough to cause the same deterioration process, and faster, of the steak left on the counter.

It should be pretty obvious that to maintain your body in good health, to stay disease-free and feeling good, you have to keep your distribution system moving with what I call "three fluffies" a day. Yes, fluffies! All my friends now call me Fluffie Schwarz.

I know, fluffies seems like an innocuous and ridiculous word for fecal matter, but it does characterize the shape and healthy condition of eliminated food from a well-functioning colon. Ideally, a meal goes in your stomach and comes out through the colon as soon as possible. Two to three fluffies a day. Yes, two to three bowel movements a day. They should be a healthy size, and they should float. What you put in your stomach has a direct impact on what comes out, and it definitely affects how you feel day by day. What are the answers to get you moving deliberately and with regularity? What are the answers to cleaning you from the inside out? There are several:

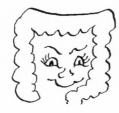

Happy
Colon

~ ~

Answer Number One: Fiber

Eat more fiber! Fiber! Fiber! Fiber! How much do you eat each day? I bet you don't know. Well, find out for your life's sake. The average American consumes about eight grams of fiber a day. The American Cancer Society and the American Heart Association agree that you should be eating between thirty and forty grams of fiber a day. Increase your fiber intake. In the countries of the world where cancer and heart disease are low people live on high-fiber diets.

The transit time for moving waste out of your body is very important. In the methodical studies done by Dr. Alexander Walker which compare transit times of waste elimination for American and African cultures, he discovered that high-fiber diets remove the waste from the intestinal system in less than half the time that it takes for low-fiber diets. To me that is a very important "life point" to know because the faster the waste passes through your body, the less time toxins have to poison your system, which can lead to disease.

Psyllium husks is one of the best fibers you can put in your body. It is eight times more fibrous than oat bran. The food most of us eat is overprocessed, and

~ ~

there is very little or no fiber in it at all. A meal at the fast-food restaurant is not a meal loaded with fiber. Junk food is typically fat food. One of the secrets to my weight-loss plan is to eat more fiber. In my own body the fiber helped clean out the fat along with everything else. So if you want to lose weight, add fiber to your diet and cut out the fat foods, and you are on your way. When you eat fiber you get full faster. Then you don't want to eat as much of the other stuff or the junk. It works! There are other important things to do that I'll talk about later, but you can tell my message, loud and clear, is to eat more fiber.

I eat a scoop of fiber (with herbs) every morning and every evening to be sure I'm getting my correct daily intake. With the lifestyle so many of us have, which doesn't always allow us to eat the way we should, we need to add fiber to our meals on a regular basis. Such regularity will assure the three-time daily frequency of your waste elimination.

Answer Number Two: Water

You can live without food, but you cannot live without water. Water is the fluid of life. Not beer, or

~ ~

wine, or orange juice, but *water!* Don't get me wrong; I enjoy a glass of wine once in a while, but most of us don't drink enough water. We aren't eating enough fiber, and we aren't drinking enough water. Now, if you will follow my example, you will change that! One of the most healthy things you can do is to drink more water. You have to do that anyway when you add more fiber to your diet because if you don't drink enough water, you will virtually stop up. Fiber adds bulk, and you need water to push it through.

How much water should you be drinking every day? I bet you know the answer to that question: eight glasses. Eight is the magic number. How can I do that, you ask? Carry a bottle of water everywhere you go. Take it with you. Get one of those water bottles and keep it filled up. Drink one glass of water after you eat each meal and drink one glass between meals and that's five glasses right there. Add one more glass when you get up in the morning. Then drink two glasses during the evening and there is the magic number of eight.

"What kind of water should I drink?" This is a question that people ask me. Well, first of all, filtered water is the best. I have a saying, "Either buy a filter or be a filter." You see. if you don't use filtered water then

~ ~

you become the filter! That means that your body has to filter out the pollutants, chemicals, toxins, and even parasites that are probably in the water you drink. You can filter or purify it in your own home with a water purifier or buy it filtered. The most important thing is to drink water. If I have to drink water out of a hotel bathroom faucet because I can't get it anywhere else at two in the morning, then that is what I drink. Better to have that water than no water at all. However, it has become a way of life for my husband and me to carry filtered bottled water with us most of the time. Count your glasses of water. That is the only way you will know that you are drinking enough. Unless you count, you can shortchange yourself. So count what you drink. Come up with a way or system to know if you truly had eight glasses a day. And remember: orange juice, beer or pop do not count. Only water counts for the eight a day!

Answer Number Three: Herbs

I love my herbs! They have changed my life more than any other single thing I have ever done to help my body. I believe that herbs are perfect food. In the Bible in Genesis 1:29, it says: "I have given you every herb

~ ~

that yields seed which is on the face of all the earth; to you it shall be for food."

Just imagine for a moment that *you* created a wonderful, beautiful being. You gave it intelligence and mobility and the ability to create. You gave it freedom of choice so it could make its own decisions, and you provided it with everything it would need to sustain its life. You also provided it with wonderful herbs and fruits and vegetables and water to help it grow and prosper. However, the being you created got off the "path" and found potato chips, mayonnaise, candy, cigarettes, alcohol and chemicals, just to name a few things. As the creator you'd probably say, "Wait a minute; you forgot about the herbs and the beautiful food I gave you so you could function at your very best."

You'd probably also be thinking, no wonder this being doesn't feel good and no wonder he is overweight and feels stressed out. "Look what he is doing to himself," you might say. Well, isn't that what happened to a lot of us? I wonder if God isn't expressing the same doubts about us as human beings. By the way, we have created wonderful beings in our children, and we have fed them the "bad stuff" as well as feeding it to ourselves. We think nothing of taking a prescription

~ ~

drug, and yet I see people cringe when they think about taking an herb in a capsule form.

The herbs have been here all along, and now many people are awakening to the miracle of herbs and what they do to move the body into perfect balance and alignment. When the body is given the right things and moves into balance, illness is not an option anymore.

There are wonderful herbs that cleanse the intestinal tract safely. There are many books where you can read about which herbs to use. I believe in the healing power of herbs. Without my herbs I know I would not be rid of the conditions that plagued me before. Just a few of the wonderful cleansing herbs are: Senna, Buckthorn, Peppermint, Orange Peel, Rose Hips, Honeysuckle Flower, Uva Ursi, and Chamomile Flower. I have also personally experienced the herb Cascara Sagrada as a powerful colon cleanser when I needed to break the dam and get the flow moving through. Another choice for me, in addition to the above-mentioned herbs, is Aloe Vera. I take an Aloe Vera capsule every morning and every evening. The Aloe is not only great for cleansing the entire gastrointestinal system but also for keeping your skin soft and supple from the inside out.

~ ~

"So, how do I cleanse my body with these herbs?" you ask. The simplest say is to drink an herbal cleansing tea every night, along with the fiber I mentioned earlier, to cleanse you inside each and every day. The herbal tea I use tastes so wonderful, and I have never been a tea drinker. Now, however, the natural cleansing tea I use has become a ritual, and I love it!

People sometimes say, "Are herbs addicting?" My response is, "No, is water addicting?" You need water, you need fiber, and you need herbs to cleanse your body on a regular basis. It is a choice. You can eat foods that stop you up or you can eat herbs (remember, herbs are food) that keep you moving and clean inside. The choice is up to you. For me, there is no choice at all.

3

Three Concepts for Body Wellness

~ ~ ~ ~ ~ ~ ~ ~ ~ ~ ~ ~ ~ ~

The nutritionist I hired explained that there are three basic concepts associated with preparing the body for a revitalized condition that will lead to a feeling of complete health and well-being.

Here are the concepts and how they work to strengthen the body and give it remarkable energy:

Concept Number One: Cleaning House
or
Cleaning Your Body from the Inside Out

What a concept! I'd never thought about it. Have you ever thought about it? Think about all the stuff you

~ ~

put inside your body and what that can do to "dirty" up your system. As Americans, we are almost fanatical about "cleaning the outside" of our bodies. We shower every day, wash our hair, our faces, and we apply inhibitors to prevent our body odor from offending, yet we never think about cleaning the inside of ourselves. If you spread butter, margarine, potato chips, fudge, bacon, mayonnaise, and peanut butter all over the outside of you, you would be clamoring in no time at all to wash it off. We complain about the smoke from cigarettes or too much alcohol, or herbicides and pesticides in our food. We try to avoid the candida (yeast) caused from antibiotics and molds, the pollutants in the air that we breathe, and the parasites (yes, parasites) living in the meat, pork, and water that we put into our bodies. Yet we put this stuff inside our bodies and think nothing of it. Think about the erosive effect of these things in your veins, arteries, blood, and intestinal tract. There are things floating around in your organs that would freak you out if you could see them. The plaque that builds up inside can kill people and does.

So, having imparted this information to me, the nutritionist said, "Barb, we are going to cleanse the inside of you."

~ ~

Concept Number Two: Burning the Fuel
or
Burning the Fat in Your Body
the Healthy Way

Since some kinds of fat are bad, but not all of them, my nutritionist said certain kinds of fat in my body should be eliminated. She pointed out that everyone needs some fat in his or her body. There are good fats and bad fats. For many of us, though, the bad fats seem to have taken over. The bad ones are the highly polyunsaturated fats and the hydrogenated fats. They are the worst fats of all. The good fats are found in the omega 3 fats and oils like canola oil or flaxseed oil. Even if you are not overweight, I suggest that you read this section, as it will help you stay thin and healthy. If you are overweight, you should definitely read on.

As you get older, your body metabolism traditionally slows down. Part of that is because even though you may be "busy," you probably are not doing the physical exercise that you once did. Everybody's body is different! It is true that what does work for one may not work for another. However, I have found that the following steps have worked for almost everyone: Clean

~ ~

the inside of your body (as described above), eat a low-fat diet, consume herbs that burn up the fat, get the "right" kind of exercise for yourself, and adopt a PMA (Positive Mental Attitude).

Eliminate Foods with Fat, Sugar, and Salt from Your Daily Diet.

I know it is not always easy, yet it is so important to cut as much fat, sugar, and salt out of your meals as possible. You have heard this advice before; it is not new. And when you finally make up your mind to do it, you will see pounds come off. Eat the whole-grain foods, fresh fruits and vegetables, herbs, fiber, and water. If approximately 50 percent of your foods are in whole grain, pastas, and carbohydrates, 40 percent in fresh fruits and vegetables, and 10 percent in proteins and meats, you will stay trim and slim.

Cut out the fat now! Remember, it is not the pasta that is fattening, it is what you put on it that counts. The same is true for the potato.

Use Natural Supplements to Help Burn the Fat.

I hate yo-yo dieting! You take pounds off and then you gain back more than you lost. Hence, yo-yo dieting. As you probably know, when you "diet," your body

~ ~

thinks you are being starved. Your brain says, "Oh, we are having a famine, so when it is time to eat again (after this diet), we'd better eat more to get ready for the next famine." That's what it says. No wonder you gain back more than you lost. Once again, herbs come to the rescue. They are so great for losing weight. I think of them as "herbal liposuction." They go to where the fat is and suck it out. And, since herbs are perfect food, your body knows what to do with them. Sometimes you need to experiment to find the right herbal combination for you; however, that is not hard to do, and it is worth the small time it takes to find the right ones.

Here are a few of the herbs, minerals, fibers, amino acids, and enzymes that I have successfully used myself to release (lose) the weight and keep it off forever:

Herbs, Fibers, Enzymes, and Minerals That Help Burn Fat

Kelp is a wonderful herb for losing weight. It is a natural diuretic and is also great for the thyroid gland.

Chromium is a trace mineral that helps your body balance its blood sugar. Because of the way farming is done today many Americans are Chromium deficient.

~ ~

Chinese Ephedra (not to be confused with the synthetic drug Ephedrine) is an herb that helps convert body fat into energy. It assists your body in burning up fat, aiding thermogenesis in your body. Two of your body's pathways are the fat pathway and the energy pathway. Ephedra helps direct fat into the energy pathway. It has been safely used by the Chinese people for more than five thousand years. If you have health challenges check with a qualified health practitioner before using Ephedra.

Garcinia Cambogia is a Southeast Asian herb that helps block your body's ability to convert complex carbohydrates and sugars into fat via the liver. Avoid alcoholic beverages at least two hours before or after taking Garcinia Cambogia, as alcohol neutralizes the effectiveness of the Garcinia Cambogia. Alcohol is one of the worst things (coffee being another one) to drink when you want to lose weight.

Glycine and *L-Methionine* can help remove fat from your liver. In addition, these amino acids with herbs will help suppress your appetite for foods high in fats. If your liver is overloaded, you've got to get it cleansed to lose weight. Burdock is another wonderful herb to cleanse the liver, as well as one called Blessed Thistle.

~ ~

Carnitine is produced by the liver. It is an amino acid. Although a supplement cannot replace exercise, it can really help burn fat. If you want to lose weight and have more energy, use a Carnitine supplement. I drink a Carnitine energy drink every day, and it works. The drink also has lots of B vitamins, bee pollen, potassium, niacin and calcium in it! I don't snack between meals when I drink this wonderful source of energy.

ଓ ଓ ଓ

By the way, cut out the coffee. I haven't had a cup of coffee for over eight years! I don't miss it one bit. You see, caffeine interferes with your metabolism, and you won't lose the weight because it is so much harder for your body to burn the fat when you drink coffee or pop. Caffeine can overstimulate your adrenal glands as well. I drink my Carnitine drink instead, and people are always amazed when they are around me. I have so much energy that they think I drink coffee, and when I tell them I don't, then they want what I drink. When you make the switch you won't get the coffee jitters anymore.

Chitosan is a natural product that is created from the exoskeletons of shrimp or crab. It is a fiber that has

~ ~

no calories, and it binds with fat and prevents it from being absorbed by the body. Then it, along with the fats, are expelled out of your body! This is truly exciting! Just think of it: Chitosan absorbs and binds the fats so you won't! Not only does it promote weight loss, but it also lowers the bad cholesterol and boosts the good cholesterol. It is antibacterial and acts as an antacid. Chitosan also helps to prevent constipation and is known to strengthen bones as it is a calcium enhancer. This is one great discovery. I eat it in capsule form with my lunch and my dinner. It does not know the good fats from the bad fats, so I do not use it with my breakfast when I take my vitamin E supplement, because if I did it would remove the vitamin E support from my body.

Concept Number Three: Building the Temple or Building Your Body with Natural Supplements

A great concept is the idea of building your body from the inside out! I have a saying, and that is: "Think right, eat right, exercise right, sleep right, and supplement right!"

~ ~

Supplement, supplement, supplement! In addition to my meals, I supplement my body in the following five main ways:

1. Natural Vitamins. I said natural. Many of the supplements you can buy are synthetic. Be sure you use natural vitamins. Your body knows what to do with natural. Of course, some of the most important vitamins are the A's, B's, C's, D's and E's.

2. Minerals. We are mineral deficient in this country! When you take the natural vitamins, it is important to take minerals at the same time. Your body cannot absorb the vitamins without the minerals present. The minerals help your body absorb the vitamins, so take a good natural vitamin/mineral combination. Some of the most important minerals to add to your diet are Calcium, Magnesium, Zinc, Selenium, and Potassium. Calcium alone is a super mineral. It is believed and reported that calcium may help prevent heart disease, ease menstrual woes, help you avoid kidney stones, and help fight osteoporosis. When taking the minerals it is best to use a chelated powdered form so that your body can absorb them and not just pass them unused out through your system. For the different minerals I use every day, I take them in powdered or

~ ~

liquid form. If you use a liquid, be sure it is in ionic form, as that will be absorbed immediately into your bloodstream. Some people think a colloidal form of liquid mineral is the best, but that has to be broken down to the ionic form in your stomach to be absorbed anyway. So I use an ionic form to begin with.

3. Fiber. We have already talked about how important fiber is. Be sure to add fiber every day to your schedule.

4. Antioxidants. The use of this word is relatively new. To put you in the picture, think of your insides as rusting as you get older. This is due to the effect of oxygen. Yet, we need oxygen to breathe and live even though it ages us, and the pollution in the air damages our cells. In addition to pollution in the air, there are many things that can damage our cells: stress, cigarette smoke (primary and secondhand), chlorine in the water, poor diets, alcohol, herbicides, pesticides, smog, certain fats, certain prescription drugs, and so on.

When a cell is damaged and loses an electron, it is called a free radical. An antioxidant, when consumed, can actually donate one of its electrons to help the free radical become a whole cell again. If unaddressed, a free radical takes an electron from a vital cell structure,

~ ~

damaging the cell and eventually causing disease. Damage from free radicals is thought to contribute to the aging process, and research suggests this damage may contribute to coronary disease, cancer rates, cataracts, MS, lupus, arthritis, and other diseases as well.

So you can see why I am so excited about antioxidants. At one time the bark of pine trees was thought to have the highest level of antioxidants in it. I used to bow before pine trees and take a bite. (No, I'm just kidding.) Today, however, it is the seeds of grapes that are thought to have the highest levels. And here we have been spitting them out all this time. Now you can hardly even buy grapes with seeds in them. I take an antioxidant in capsule form every morning. The bioflavonoids found in grape seed have been so wonderful for my health and for my family's health. Some people remark about how great my skin looks, and I think that is one of the reasons why. *I love my antioxidants!* I'm out to get the world on them. Some of the other important antioxidants include vitamin E, vitamin A, Selenium, and coenzyme Q_{10}.

5. Herbs. I know you can tell by now how much I believe in and love herbs. You will too! Begin by using a few, and then experiment a little and determine as you

~ ~

add others which ones seem to work in your body the best. I eat about thirty to forty different herbs a day. I know that sounds like a lot, but it's not. I have never looked better or felt better in my life.

When was the last time you had thirty to forty potato chips? I bet it wasn't that long ago, and if you did eat them you may not have thought anything about doing it. I eat my herbs in less time than it would take for you to eat those chips, and I know you know which is better for you. I rest my case. You could eat the herbs straight out of a baggie that you bought from an herbalist like I used to eat them, but some of them don't taste very good. Now I eat them in capsules. It takes less time, less work, and I don't have to taste them when they are going down. I have not been sick once since I have been on "my herbs"!

I believe that herbs move the body into healing. Here are some of my favorite ones and what they have done for the body historically:

Herbs That Build: Historical Uses

Aloe Vera. Promotes healing of skin, stomach and the colon. Helpful with constipation.

~ ~

Black Cohosh. Helps regulate menstrual flow and menstrual cramps, balances hormones, strengthens heart and lungs, works as a relaxant.

Black Walnut. Fights infection, cleanses parasites, burns fat, helps to regulate blood sugar levels.

Blue Vervain. Useful for colds, promotes sweating, increases circulation, helps in healing of liver and bowels.

Bilberry. Rich in manganese, which improves eyesight; used for night blindness.

Cascara Sagrada. Natural and safe herbal laxative; kills harmful bacteria in the intestines and colon, helpful for high blood pressure.

Cayenne. Works as a catalyst for other herbs; very helpful with colds and flu; helpful with heart, strokes and controlling cholesterol.

Dandelion. Rich in minerals; helpful for digestive tract and liver; removes toxins.

Devil's Claw. Natural cleanser; helps reduce kidney and liver problems; useful for arthritis; promotes flexibility in joints.

Dong Quai. Very helpful for the female challenges of PMS, menopause; stabilizes blood sugar levels; dissolves blood clots.

~ ~

Echinacea. Fights infection and virus; sinus infections; boosts the immune system; may be helpful with Lyme disease, Addison's disease, Legionnaires' disease, tuberculosis, and AIDS. Echinacea is known as nature's antibiotic.

Garlic. Kills infection and parasites; kills candida yeast; builds immune system.

Ginseng. Known as the King of Herbs; improves concentration and memory; improves circulation; promotes overall well-being; may be helpful with ADD and also with AIDS.

Goldenseal. Helpful with mucus membranes; relieves cold and flu symptoms; mouthwash for gum disease; anti-inflammatory.

Gotu Kola. Known as the "memory herb"; used with stress, depression and mental challenges; historically helpful with schizophrenia, epilepsy, ADD, and anorexia. Relaxes the nerves and strengthens the heart.

Hawthorn Berries. Wonderful for the whole cardiovascular system; helps prevent hardening of the arteries; regulates blood pressure.

Licorice. Used by the Chinese for over 5,000 years; helpful with throat conditions, female problems, hypo-

~ ~

glycemia; increases energy. May raise blood pressure in some people.

Lobelia. Used as a relaxant; helps to loosen mucus; used for asthma, migraine headaches, allergies, and has a wonderful effect on the whole body.

Passion Flower. Used for stress — very relaxing; helps with menopause; relaxant for coughs; used for muscle twitching. High in calcium.

Pau d'Arco. Wonderful for the whole body; anti-tumor and anti-fungal; kills viruses; builds immune system. Helpful perhaps with lupus, diabetes, asthma, arthritis, and liver challenges. Overall effective herb.

Red Clover. Cleanses and purifies the blood; fights cancerous growths; reported to be helpful with cancer, lupus, AIDS, muscle atrophy, psoriasis, other skin problems, and Lyme disease.

Red Raspberry. High in minerals and vitamins; overall female tonic; good for stomach and intestinal tract.

Slippery Elm. Wonderful for constipation and hemorrhoids; helps kidney problems; soothes mucous membranes; helpful for the whole body.

Suma. Helps the adrenaline glands; used to help fight stress and fatigue; menopause; perhaps helpful with Lyme disease and AIDS.

~ ~

Valerian. Used to reduce tension and anxiety; helpful with insomnia, heart palpitations, arthritis, high blood pressure, and headaches.

Wild Yam. Used for nervousness, female challenges, cramps and spasms; this is a very soothing herb.

Yellow Dock. Builds the immune system and balances the body's chemistry.

ဢ ဢ ဢ

The herbs I've listed are certainly not all of the herbs available to you or me by any stretch of the imagination. These are just some of my favorites, ones I have used the longest. To bring my body into balance, I traditionally use herbal combinations for the greatest impact. There are many different kinds of herbal combinations. I have my favorite herbal recipes and combinations that have helped me and others with all kinds of challenges. There is simply not enough room in this book to go into the benefits of all of them. When I think of building the temple of the body, I also think about several other things which I would like you to be aware of, things which have made such a difference in my life:

~ ~

Melatonin. Melatonin naturally exists in our bodies, and as we age our bodies produce less. Research shows it is perfectly safe to add a small dose of melatonin at bedtime. Some of the benefits include: lowering of blood pressure and the normalizing of cholesterol. It eases stress, is a nonaddictive and potent sleeping aid, and strengthens the immune system and helps raise the body's resistance to cancer and other diseases such as heart disease.

CO-Q_{10}. CO-Q_{10} is a co-enzyme. Your cells need this nutrient for energy. Research indicates that CO-Q_{10} can heal periodontal problems, protect against heart attack, boost the immune system, slow the aging process, lower high blood pressure, and possibly extend life. Your body naturally makes CO-Q_{10} out of other co-enzymes, or you can absorb it from foods. But as you age, your body may produce less, and it is hard to depend on foods for CO-Q_{10} because it is lost with processing and storage. I use supplementation of CO-Q_{10} daily for all of these reasons!

Glucosamine. Glucosamine is a lifesaver for people with arthritis and joint degeneration. Use glucosamine as a dietary supplement. Research shows it will help the body build more cartilage. Glucosamine signals the

~ ~

body to stop destroying cartilage and to help rebuild it, and it stimulates the body's manufacture of collagen which is the protein portion of the body's connective tissue.

Summary

When I think of wellness, body balance, and vitality, I always think about these three major concepts I've listed:

Concept Number One: Cleaning House:
   Cleaning your body from the inside out

Concept Number Two: Burning the Fuel:
   Burning the fat in your body the healthy way

Concept Number Three: Building the Temple:
   Building your body with natural supplements.

⅋ ⅋ ⅋

~ ~

This program keeps me healthy, fit, vitally alive, and full of energy. These concepts will work for you too! Remember, "Ask not what your body can do for you, but what you can do for your body."

~ ~

4

Not in Our House

~ ~ ~ ~ ~ ~ ~ ~ ~ ~ ~ ~ ~ ~

The real voyage of discovery consists not in seeking new landscapes but in having new eyes.

– Jonathan Swift

This chapter is a lifesaver! Use it as a reference when you are shopping or eating out. Keep the foods listed out of your body as much as possible. We try not to keep these foods in our house at all. If we do, it is only for a short time. If you don't bring them home, then you won't eat them. Remember, it isn't what you do from Hanukkah or Christmas to New Year's that counts,

~ ~

but rather what you do from New Year's to Hanukkah or Christmas that really matters.

When my husband Kirk and I go to see the Sonics play basketball in Seattle, the crowd always shouts, "Not in Our House," when they don't like the thought of losing. Applying the slogan to your body will keep you away from harmful foods. Stay away from those described in this chapter as much as you can.

Thirteen Foods and Preservatives to Avoid

1. Fast Food. Fast food is usually fat food. We have been raising American children on fast food. No wonder there are more obese children in our country than ever before. Limit your intake of fast food and restrict the amount of fast food for your children.

2. Sodium Nitrate Meats. Stay away from meats that have sodium nitrates in them. Sodium nitrates cause cancer in rats. This means limit your intake of bacon, pepperoni, hot dogs, salami, bologna, and ham. The University of Southern California School of Medicine in Los Angeles found that youngsters eating more than twelve hot dogs a month had nearly ten times the risk of developing leukemia as the kids who ate none. Other

~ ~

evidence from the University of North Carolina shows children eating nitrite-cured meats had an 80 percent higher risk of brain cancer. A Dutch study of men and women showed increased colon cancer risk when it came to sausage because of the nitrate curing agents in it. Restrict sodium nitrate meats in your body!

3. Fake Sugar. One of the packages of fake sugar says right on the envelope that it is known to cause cancer in laboratory animals. Fake sugar messes up the natural balance of your body. In some people it causes headaches, nausea, stomach upset, diarrhea, and allergy problems. If you have to add something for sweetener, use pure raw honey, or maple syrup.

4. Caffeine. America is caffeine-addicted. Caffeine is a drug. It causes the blood vessels in your brain to swell. This is one of the reasons you get headaches when you try to get off caffeine. Coffee increases the heart attack risk in men by 50 percent. Wean yourself off of coffee, pop and chocolate. They are all loaded with caffeine.

5. Shellfish/Bottom Fish. Bottom fish eat the waste of other fish on the bottom of the sea. Our oceans are becoming so polluted with arsenic, mercury and lead that it is wise to stay away from shellfish and bottom

~ ~

fish for this reason. When it comes to fish, the best ones to eat are salmon, tuna, mackerel, sardines, and herring because they have the most antiaging omega-3 fatty acids in them.

6. *Dairy Products.* Many allergy problems come from dairy products. Part of the problem is the high fat content in many dairy products. Why are we the only animals that continue to eat and drink dairy products after we have been weaned from our mothers? Interesting food for thought, huh?

7. *Alcohol.* Just three ounces of alcohol can decrease your body's ability to digest fat by 30 percent. Alcohol is fattening in itself, and it also interferes with your body's metabolism. Limit your alcohol. Drink red wine if you drink because it has more antioxidants in it than white wine.

8. *Mayonnaise.* Mayonnaise is 100 percent fat. All of its calories come from fat. I always say mayonnaise causes "blood sludge."

9. *Margarine.* This clogs the pores. I think of coronary glue when I think of margarine. Hydrogenated fats are found in margarines. You are better off using real butter than margarine. The best is to not use either. Use almost exclusively olive oil, canola oil, or

~ ~

macadamia nut oil. These are much better choices for cooking. When it comes to eating bread, get used to the taste of the bread by itself. Buy whole-grain or nine-grain breads and you will begin to taste how great it really is. Whenever I am tempted to reach for the margarine or the butter, I just imagine a jar of Vaseline sitting on the table, because there is no more nutrition in margarine or butter than there is in Vaseline for your body.

10. Chlorine. Filter your water. Chlorine elevates the LDL cholesterol levels in your body. Colon and uterine cancers have increased, research shows, since chlorine has been added to water. There are many units you can purchase to filter your water at home. You can attach one to your faucet or buy a water pitcher that has a built-in filter in it.

11. Sugar Snacks. They'll take you for a ride. One minute they'll give you energy, and the next they'll put you on the floor. Your blood sugar goes for a joy ride, and you may end up a wreck. Someone once asked me, "How can a two-pound box of candy make you gain five pounds?" Good question, isn't it? So, use natural snacks for an energy boost, not snacks that are loaded with sugar.

~ ~

12. Fats. Meat, dairy products like cheese, poultry skin, salad dressings, ice cream, candy (the list goes on) are all high sources of fat. Learn to read the labels on the things you buy at the store. Look at the fat grams and the percentage of fat in the processed food you take home with you. These days I believe the fat intake is more important to watch than the total number of calories you are putting into your body. It is the high percentage of calories from fat that is the real problem in the search for better health. Become a fat stopper.

13. MSG. Stay away from eating foods that have MSG added to them. Do not use it in your cooking or food preparation at home either. It is addictive and causes allergy problems for many people.

Also, limit your intake of meat. Trim fat from the meat you do eat and take the skin off the poultry. Read labels. Make your own fat-free dressings. Cookbooks are full of fat-free recipes today. Find the ones you like and stick with them, and then share them with others you care about. You know the first thing a doctor says when there is a heart problem is to cut out fat. Don't wait until a doctor tells you that. Do it now!

~ ~

"What Can I Eat?"

You may say, "Well, if I stay away
from all these foods, what can I eat?
There is nothing left." Sorry, that is
just not true. There are all kinds of
great foods left to eat. For
beginners, start with fresh foods.
Fresh fruits and fresh vegetables. Eat
whole grains, fish, nuts, legumes,
soybeans, potatoes, rice, and pastas.
Remember, it isn't the pasta that puts on weight, it's
what you put on it that can cause the problem, so no
cream sauces. Here is some of the "good stuff" to put in
your body at any time:

The Good Stuff in Our House

Garlic	Broccoli	Kelp
Avocado	Cauliflower	Grapefruit
Brussels Sprouts	Asparagus	Potatoes
Tomatoes	Cantaloupe	Alfalfa
Oat Bran	Grains	Figs
Beets	Dates	Cabbage
Radishes	Cucumbers	Artichokes

~ ~

Parsley	Pears	Kiwi
Papaya	Guava	Nectarines
Apricots	Blackberries	Plums
Cherries	Tangerines	Peaches
Onions	Zucchini	Carrots
Spinach	Pumpkin	Squash
Peppers	Pineapples	Watermelon
Melons	Strawberries	Grapes
Oranges	Apples	Okra
Sprouts	Beans	Rice
Soybeans	Legumes	Brazil Nuts
Psyllium Husks	Canola Oil	Olive Oil
Selected Poultry	Good Fish	Herbs
Herbs	Herbs	Herbs!

The most important decision of all is to eat more fresh fruits and vegetables. Buy more fruits and vegetables. They are loaded with antioxidants which your body needs to keep you young, healthy and glowing, and then look for interesting ways to prepare them. Go to the organically grown section of your store and eat your fill. Aren't you bored at the grocery store anyway? It's time to branch out. Live it up. Have a ball. Learn to cook all over again. We did. I've learned to cook all

~ ~

kinds of tasty, healthy, different dishes. Have fun, eat right, and keep the bad stuff away from your home. Remember: "Not in Our House!"

~ ~

Your Mind

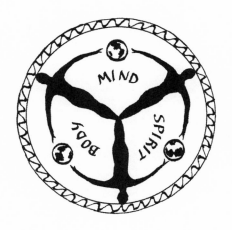

5

Empowering Your Mind
to Create the Life You Want

~ ~ ~ ~ ~ ~ ~ ~ ~ ~ ~ ~ ~ ~

The attacker is not out there, but within.
– Morihei Ueshiba

Everyone thinks of changing the world, but
no one thinks of changing themselves.
– Tolstoy

You can create the life you want. Educating your mind and controlling your thoughts are two major keys to creating the life you desire. Before we look at the steps to making the life you want, let's look at some simple but effective statements which will empower you

~ ~

by providing a strong foundation and keep you on the right track:

- Your brain is a muscle. Exercise it every day.
- Keep an open mind. Your mind is like a parachute: it can't work if it isn't open.
- Educate your mind.
- Know that you can control your thoughts.
- Practice controlling your thoughts.
- Rid your mind of negativity.
- When you think a thought that brings you down, do what my thirteen-year-old friend Jeffrey Altenburg does. He simply says to himself, "Erase that!" It's just that easy! Then replace the negative thought with a positive one immediately.
- Give up worry. Don't consume your mind with it. It is interest on a loan that hardly ever comes due.
- Live in the moment. Enjoy the now.
- Thoughts and words have incredible power. The power of thoughts actually can be measured.
- Thoughts are energy in motion. Choose your thoughts; it is your mind!

જી જી જી

~ ~

Most of us do not understand how the brain works, but there is one aspect which, if you understand it, can help you immeasurably to achieve your goals in life. This one aspect is the fact that the brain cannot distinguish between reality and imagination. The mind, by giving the brain instructions, can actually alter brain cells, enabling the body to perform an imagined result.

A classic case of mind over matter was reported by Michael Murphy and Rhea White in their book, *In the Zone*. They wrote about an angler, Richard Reinwald, who imagined a trophy-winning fish, then proceeded to catch the California state record brown trout. He picked Flaming Gorge to fish in and told many people in the nearby town of Bishop that he would hook the record fish. "Every day I actually pictured the record fish in my mind," he wrote.... "The picture was clear as a bell, a hen fish, the colors rather dark." And that is what he caught, a female brown trout darker than the others he had been catching.

The famous physiologist Sir John Eccles made the same proposal. In an invited address at the 1976 convention of the Parapsychological Association, he proposed that the simple act of saying a word was actually a form of psychokinesis: "The mind has been able to work

~ ~

upon the brain cells, just slightly changing them.... The mind is making these very slight and subtle changes for hundreds of millions of cells, gradually bringing the impulse through and channeling it into the correct target cells to make the movement. And so there is psycho-kinesis, mind acting upon a material object, namely brain cells. It's extremely weak, but it's effective, because we've learned to use it."

I suggest that we all have the ability to extend the health of the body beyond the confines of the flesh. But where does this energy come from? I believe it's from God, the Universe, the ultimate power source, which, if we use our minds wisely, we can tap.

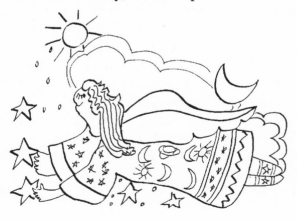

~ ~

Steps to Creating the Life You Want

Your life is a canvas. You can create whatever you like. If it feels as though your life is out of balance, you can choose in an instant to begin again. The following steps will help you use your mind, together with your spirit, as a power center. If you do not understand the steps, that is okay; practice them anyway. The more you say them and affirm them, the more they will be a part of you, and the more you will create what you want in your life. I have found in my own life that the steps work. It is true that whatever you can conceive and believe you will achieve. Remember, the brain cannot distinguish between imagination and reality. Learn the steps, know them, and use them daily.

Step One:
Believe in the Power of the Universe

There is but one force, one power, one intelligence, one presence, and one consciousness moving through this Universe. It is omnipotent and omnipresent. It is in everything. As you recognize that God is, it immediately elevates your conscious mind to the spiritual level. This fills you with confidence, it excites

~ ~

you, and it relaxes you all at the same time. Believing in the power of the Universe and God opens you up to all the good that follows, and it supports you only as truth can.

> *If you knew who walks beside you on the way that you have chosen, fear would be impossible.*
>
> *– The Course in Miracles*

Step Two:
Believe the Universal Power Is in You

> *The currents of the universal being circulate through me; I am part and parcel of God.*
>
> *– Ralph Waldo Emerson*

Because God is, God is in you. God is not just "out there." God is on the inside of you. You are a crucial part of this Universe. There is a reason you are here. Know and believe that the same energy and power of the sun and the stars is in you.

Most people feel separated from God. That is the reason we separate ourselves from each other. If God seems far away, guess *who* moved! Every problem we

~ ~

have on this planet comes from separating ourselves from our source and from each other. The dilemma is not that we are separate from God, but that we think we are separate from God. All we need to do is change our belief.

Step Three:
Believe That What You Desire
Already Exists

Ninety-nine percent of who you are is invisible and untouchable.
– Buckminster Fuller

Know that you can create and have what you desire in your life. Simply ask and believe. That means that you ask and believe that it already exists and that it will "show up" at the right time in the right way for you and for your highest good. You accept it in "mind" and it will appear. This is an action step. I do not know how it works. I don't need to know how it works. I just know it works. Some people spend so much time trying to figure out the "how" that they never get to the "do."

~ ~

I find that if I think "my time," what I desire to create seems to take longer to appear. But when I release my vision and goals to the Universe and I trust in "universal time," what I ask for always appears. This requires believing and trusting. State what your goal is in the present, as though it has already happened, and the good will appear.

Example: I am earning $ ____ or more a month as a distributor with _____. I help people create perfect health and well-being through the miracle of herbs. I help people build their own successful home-based business. I am debt free and I have abundance in all areas of my life.

Notice that I did not say "I wish" or "I want." I said "I am." If you say "I wish" or "I want," it sounds as if you think it may not happen. Always state "I am" when you are declaring to the Universe what your intentions are. It sets the achievable into motion. The other tip is to always leave your good open. Always say, "or more," when stating your desires and

~ ~

expectations. God has more good in mind for you and for me than we can ever fully imagine.

Step Four:
Be Thankful for Everything in Your Life

Learn to be thankful for everything in your life. Yes, everything. There are blessings in everything that happens to you and to me. Look for the good. As you receive good, be thankful. Thanksgiving brings abundance. Giving brings abundance, so give and share. Think about it: giving and receiving are one and the same. It is all a part of the same energy flow. Be thankful on both counts. Be thankful for the things that you know are already on their way to you. Be thankful for what you believe already exists for you. The laws of the Universe are really simple in the end:

- Believe in the Universal Power,
- Know that that Power, God, is in you,
- State your desires in the present as though they already exist,
- Expect, and accept the good you want in your life,
- Be thankful for everything in your life, and
- Release ... Let Go, Let God.

~ ~

Step Five: Release

Release, just release. This is the final act of faith. Turn it over to the Universe and go about your life with assurance that wonderful things are taking place. If you can dream it, you can create it. Let go and let God. This is the way it works: As you believe you ask. As you ask you trust. As you trust you are thankful. As you are thankful you release and let God and the Universe go to work for you and with you.

I have always believed in goal-setting. I have set goals for years. Yet, as I have discovered these steps and put them to work in my life, I have seen far greater good come my way and come to others. I have a large tablet where I write things down ... my feelings, ideas, and thoughts. I write my goals there as well. I have a page that is marked, "Things I am working on." I also have a page that is entitled, "Things that God and the Universe are Working on for Me." My page is getting shorter and shorter. God and the Universe's page is getting longer and longer. On the top of the page in my tablet is written: Things God and the Universe are Working on for Me.

~ ~

*God created me to prosper for I am a part
of the abundant Universe*

Whenever I say these words I get a burst of joy on the inside of me.

See if you don't feel the goosebumps, the "Godbumps," inside you when you say these two affirmations. The reason they feel so good and the reason you get the goosebumps is because deep down inside you, your very being knows they are true.

~ ~

Your Spirit

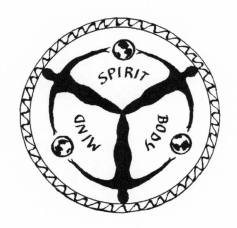

6

The Flavor of Life:
Awakening the Spirit Within

~ ~ ~ ~ ~ ~ ~ ~ ~ ~ ~ ~ ~ ~

There is a story told by spiritual leaders about the masters, who were trying to decide where to hide the most powerful force in the Universe, the ability to create miracles, so that man would never discover it until he was mature enough not to misuse it. They talked about putting it at the bottom of the deepest sea or at the top of the highest mountain, but they argued these hiding places were not perfect. Finally, they came across the perfect hiding place: they would secret it within the heart of man, because that would be the last place we would ever think to look.

~ ~

To awaken the spirit within you takes much effort, but it is worthwhile, for once you understand who you are, you will discover a Universe of knowing that is wider than the heart is wide and higher than the soul can reach. You will understand that you are not a body with a spirit. You are a spirit with a body. There is a difference. As I give my seminars and speak across the country, people ask me, "How do I tap into my spirit? How do I learn to hear it? How do I know it is there?"

Oh, it's there, all right. You would not be alive without it. You and I are energy, very special forms of energy. We are a part of the divine energy, the divine creativity of the Universe. It is in you and it is in me. Your spirit is your "higher" self, that part of you that is the expression of God. By the way, as we talk about spirit, if that word bothers you, replace it with any word you feel more comfortable with. Whether you say spirit, God, energy, universal wisdom, or mustard seed, it doesn't matter. It is all the same. Use the word that works best for you. For me it is the word spirit/God.

When I speak of your higher self, I am referring to that perfect place in you. It is that place of love and pureness inside you. In a higher sense it is the pureness and the love in which you were created. It is truly "the God" in you. Spirit is in you. God is spirit. God is in you. God is in everything. How could you be a creation on this planet, and you are, without the creator being a part, actually at the core, of who you are?

You see, your spirit connects you with all of creation and all living things. Your spirit is the link to the entire creative process. The most important thing in our definition of spirit is to understand and recognize that spirit fulfills an essential need for humankind. There is truly something in all of us that aspires to the spiritual.

That is because the spiritual awakens and inspires us as human beings because as human beings we are in the act of becoming.

Through contact with your spirit you can truly begin to value all life forms and the flow of life. You will find yourself releasing fears from your life, and you will begin to live in the moment, as you grow to appreciate everything life has to offer us. At that point healing begins.

~ ~

Spiritual Growth

There are four stages of spiritual growth that are possible for us to go through. Many people find themselves mired in the early "victim" stage, though at times we may glimpse the purity of the most advanced stage in which yearning and completion meld together. Which stage are you in? Sometimes you may vacillate back and forth from one stage to the next. The goal is Stage Number Four, the most advanced stage of peace and knowing. That is where you live through your creative self. That is where you tap into the power of the Universe to work for you to bring you whatever you desire in your life.

Stage One: The Victim

This stage is where you feel the world is happening "to you." You feel you are a "victim" of everything around you. You feel your spouse is doing things to you. You think your mother is ruining your life. You feel victim to the economic strains of the country. You are convinced your company has made your life miserable. And on and on and on. In other words, you feel the world is out to "get you," and you think that

~ ~

there is nothing you can do about it. Yes, you are a victim because you think you are. This is a stage or state of mind in which you are totally reactive. You react to life rather than create it. Two questions to ask yourself during trying situations are:

"Am I being reactive or proactive in this situation?" and, "Am I being reactive or proactive in my life?"

If your answer to either question is reactive, then life is not as much fun for you. Fear, anger, self-doubt, and negative thoughts reign supreme here. It is like playing on the defensive side of a football team. You are always trying to figure out what the other team is going to do. You constantly react to their moves. You work hard to keep them from scoring. You feel bruised, beat up, and tired. Usually, when you are tired enough of living life as a victim you will move to the next stage of growth.

Stage Two: Ownership
(Self-Responsibility)

This is the stage of growth where you take full responsibility for your life.

~ ~

Here you leave the world of the reactive, and you take a positive stance in all areas of your life. You have come to understand that you never will be able to control other people, but you can sure control yourself. You stop blaming other people for things that happen to you and you move into your life by realizing that you do have control over your own thoughts, actions, and feelings. This is the stage of "individual responsibility," and in this stage of growth you take ownership of yourself.

At the ownership stage of life no one can make you feel insulted or upset now because you know that such feelings are a personal choice. If you want to feel insulted, go for it, but now you understand it is a choice and that is different from the victim mentality in stage one.

In this stage you begin to choose joy more often because you realize and feel the control you have over your own destiny. Therefore, you begin to choose peace more than conflict.

You begin to grow.

Stage Three: Cooperative
(Universal Responsibility)

Everything is interdependent upon everything else. All of mankind and nature is interdependent. This third stage of growth is exciting because in it lies the "Ah-Ha!" — the realization that you do need other people and all of nature in its beauty to live life to the fullest. I call this stage "Universal Responsibility."

In this stage you see the relationships in all of life. You care how your neighbor feels and how your actions affect him/her. You realize that what you think does make a difference. Since you have come to understand that thoughts are energy, can be measured, and can influence people, you consciously work to harm no one or no one thing. You reach out to others in a positive way to touch the whole.

As you grow, you are able to extend the idea represented by the title of this book from, *If You Wear Out Your Body Where Will You Live?* to, *If We Wear Out Our Planet, Where We Live?* So, you recycle. You become more aware of the pollution in the sea and you know that what you do to stop it by buying safe products has an effect on the whole, even though you are one person,

~ ~

not an army. You know that the tides need the moon and the earth needs the sun and we all need each other.

Your love of life and all living things directs your path and sets you free.

Stage Four: Let Go ... Let Spirit
Let Go ... Let God

Bliss! Sweet Bliss!!! This is the place you have been looking for. This is where peace, unconditional love, joy, and happiness are found. Here you let go of what has been, and you rise to new heights of expression and awareness. You flow with life, rather than against it.

When you reach Stage Four you know, trust, and feel there is a beautiful flow to life. You have passed through Stage Three, in which you realized everything is interdependent upon everything else, so in Stage Four you trust that everything in life is happening for the good of all concerned, no matter how it looks or how it shows up. This is the point in your life when you fully acknowledge the divine. You acknowledge the divine inside you. You acknowledge that God is and that God lives in you. You acknowledge that the power and love that created the moon and planets is in you. So you relax and become "fluid."

Stay Fluid. Stay fluid with the Universe. Move with it, not against it. Emulate water which flows above an object, below it, or through it. Say to yourself: "Stay fluid with the situations in my life." As you stay fluid you begin to see the rhythm of the universe and how truly beautiful it is. When things seem to get tough, you say and feel, "Let Go and Let God."

In this stage you live your life in a state of love. You are head over heels in love with life. You listen to your heart more than your head. You accept others around you. You may not like the actions of someone you know, and yet you see the beautiful parts of who he/she is. It is called unconditional love. You care. You know you can create the life you want and you do. Deepak Chopra, the spiritualist, calls this stage living life "in the gap." You trust that the Universe, that God,

~ ~

doesn't make mistakes and that everything in your life is working for your highest good. You believe. Because you believe, "Magic Happens."

A Meditation of Peace, Love, and Joy

Imagine that you are walking barefoot through a beautiful woods. You see trees of gorgeous size and stature. There is a path you are following that is taking you on a lovely journey. Grass is beneath your feet, and you feel it between your toes. The sky is true blue, and you hear birds singing all around you. A few powder-puff clouds dot the sky, and you feel free. The song of spring sings in your heart with great love and joy.

As you enter a clearing you see a beautiful stream in front of you. The babbling water calls to you as you walk forward and drop to your knees to touch the water. It is warm. Flowers bloom beside the stream. You see no beginning to the stream, and you see no end.

You walk into the stream, and as you do you begin to float in the water. You float on your back and embrace the blue sky as the brother to your soul. The water below you carries you on the bosom of your sister, the earth. You breathe in spirit and you breathe out love. You feel greater love than you have ever known. You are one with the trees, the sky, the water, the flowers, the birds, the earth. You feel yourself merge into one with everything around you. You are one with all. You are weightless. There are no more problems. There are no more worries. There is only love and you and creation. You reach up your hand, and as you do you feel a touch.

You feel the touch of God.

In that touch you see and remember your beauty as a person. You remember the perfection inside of you, you remember the joy and the love with which you were created. You rest in the water feeling renewed, refreshed, and reconnected with your true essence. You feel love in you and all around you. You float in the arms of bliss. You are at peace with yourself and with all others. This is a place of perfect blissful love.

When you are ready, you rise, you stand. You can return to this place inside of you

~ ~

anytime your heart desires. You walk out of the water and look towards the beautiful trees. The people you love are there waiting for you. You feel no sadness, you feel no stress. You are at peace. You walk towards them with your arms outstretched, ready to embrace them and carry the oneness and the peace and the love with you. You are not the same, and you never will be the same again. Your problems have disappeared, your troubles are gone. You are blessed, you are beautiful. It was there all along. You have reawakened your spirit.

You have touched the hand of God.

– by Barb Schwarz

As you look at the pictures of me on the following two pages you may not believe the difference. The picture of me with the short hair was taken approximately ten years ago and yet I look younger today, as you see in the other picture, than I did then. No, I have not had any plastic surgery. I am now off all of my prescriptions for allergies and asthma as I have no more symptoms. I have lost weight, and I have cured my severe constipation problem once and for all by doing what I have shared with you in this book. I am a walking testimony that the herbs work! They say a picture is worth a thousand words. I'll let the pictures do the rest of the talking for me.

~ ~

Before

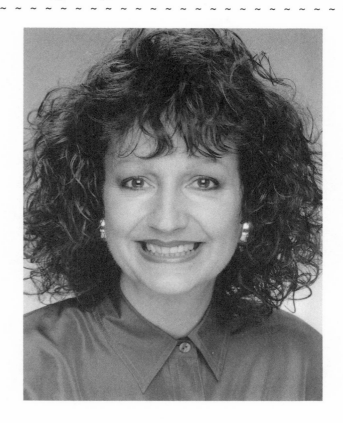

After

~ ~

7

Nourishment for the Soul: Principles for Joyous Living

~ ~ ~ ~ ~ ~ ~ ~ ~ ~ ~ ~ ~ ~

*One word frees us of all the weight and
pain of life: That word is love.*
– Sophocles, 406 B.C.

Joyous living. What wonderful words these are.
Do you believe that you can live in a state of joy? Do
you believe you can live in a place of peace in your heart
and mind? If you believe you can or if you believe you
can't, either way you are right. For the last five to seven
years, more than ever before, I have been on a conscious
journey to nourish my soul ... to feed my spirit. I have
traveled many places, read many books, and listened to

~ ~

many people. I have come to a place now where I
believe that the master is in all of us. Inside of you is a
beautiful student and a beautiful teacher. We are all
students and teachers of each other. Everything you
desire is "in you," not "out there." On my journey I have
written what I call "Principles for Joyous Living." It
gives me joy to share them with you.

Principles for Joyous Living

There are only two true emotions: one is Fear and
the other is Love. Love is spirit alive on the inside of
you; Fear is your ego at work. Ask yourself daily, "Are
the actions or steps I am about to take coming from a
place of love inside me or are they based in fear?" You
can choose love or you can choose fear as the path to
follow. If fear is your choice, then most of your actions
will be defensive; you will find yourself in a coping
state of mind rather than one of flow and peace. Accept
the fact that you are not here to ask forgiveness, but
rather to learn how to forgive.

The following are ideals for those who live for
love, apply them daily in your life:
  • Forgiveness offers you everything you want.
  • Peace is a choice.

~ ~

- Inner peace is the greatest state of health of all.
- Live in the moment. It is everything and all there really is.
- Accept others as they are; your judgments define who you are.
- Know that you are a mirror of what you see. (The things that bother you the most about others are simply mirrors of characteristics that you do not like about yourself.)
- Start accepting; stop analyzing.
- Stay "fluid" with life.
- Challenges are gifts, too.
- Live in the energy of positive thought.
- Happiness is a choice.
- Every truthful thought is love in action.
- Be your own best friend.
- Love yourself unconditionally.
- Love others unconditionally.
- Look for the love and perfect spirit on the inside of everyone you meet.
- Love is the answer.
- Abundance is a universal law.
- The Universe always says yes. Therefore, be sure you ask for what you truly want.

~ ~

- God wants you to prosper.
- The Universe wants you to be abundant.
- Abundance multiplies.
- Focus on thanksgiving.
- Realize, believe, and accept that you really are enough, just the way you are.
- Know that the greatest blessing of all is you.
- Your pure state is love; everything else is an illusion.
- Love in you is spirit expressing itself.
- Release ... Let Go ... Let God.

Your Spirit and Your Ego

As I observed earlier, love comes from your spirit, and fear comes from your ego. There are no exceptions.

The ego is a very powerful human force. Its goal is to win at all costs, no matter what. Your ego self is always trying to separate you from your real self, from who you really are. Your ego wants to rule your life. Your ego wants to control you, and many times it does by keeping you in a state of emotions based in fear. The ego's world is one of attack, pain, fear, separation, and death.

What are your fears? What are you afraid of? Are you afraid you won't make enough money? Are you afraid you won't keep your job? Are you afraid your kids won't be able to afford the "American Dream"? Are you afraid you will get sick? Are you afraid of failing? Are you afraid of success? Are you afraid to share your true deep love for yourself and for others?

Following are two columns in which Spirit and Ego are characterized by their opposites. Read these words and see where you fit.

Spirit	*Ego*
Your Pure Center	Victim Thought
Your Energy Field	System
Love	Fear
Peace	Conflict
Wellness	Illness
Present	Past
Forgiveness	Judgment
Abundance	Lack
Joining Together	Separation
Faith	Worry
Acceptance	Rejection
Responsibility	Denial
Happiness	Depression
Trust	Suspicion

~ ~

Defenseless	Defensive
Creativity	Suppression
Commitment	Procrastination
Proactive	Reactive

You see, your ego analyzes and your spirit accepts.

When you live your life from your spirit center, your life becomes so much easier. By moving to a place of love, the answers come so much easier. Yes, of course, you think about the challenge, but the answers come when you release the solution to spirit. Simply let go. Why continue to beat yourself up? When you finally do let go, you begin to feel such a freedom that you wonder why you didn't let go a long time ago.

Remember: positive emotions are based in love (spirit), and all negative emotions are based in fear (ego). When you feel threatened it is because your ego has you thinking you aren't in control in some area of your life. However,

~ ~

when you move from the spiritual center of your being and come from your heart, truthful answers always start to appear. These are the answers that work. The struggle is simply gone. Trust, faith, peace, thanksgiving, joy, and resolution replace the agony. You have now invited your spirit into the managerial role, and the intelligence of the Universe is there for the asking. Did you know that your heart has 2.5 watts of power? Research shows that the heart's electrical system is actually forty times stronger than the brain's electrical system. The electromagnetic field in the heart is a blending of love and wisdom.

Love is all intelligence. It is all powerful. It is all knowing. When you experience that ... you have experienced the link that bonds the entire universe together as one. That's what universe means. It means "one song."

Practice the Principles for Joyous Living.
Read them every day.
Learn them.
Teach them to others.
They are nourishment for the soul.

8

Kids are People Too!
Time, Love and Tenderness

~ ~ ~ ~ ~ ~ ~ ~ ~ ~ ~ ~ ~ ~

This chapter is about our children. If you have children or grandchildren, I'm sure they are the extra-special loves of your life. They are truly gifts from God. I know that is what my daughter Andrea is to me.

As we look at awakening the spirit within; empowering our minds and building our bodies, we must look at doing the same for our children. There is an old saying that goes like this: "To know and not to do is not to know." The world is moving very quickly these days and people are being pulled in all kinds of directions and that includes our children.

~ ~

Our children, right along with us, see and hear changes on our planet instantly through the power of television. That includes war, famine, crime, and violence. Our schools are overcrowded and under-staffed. Kids today are being raised on fast food; and the family unit is stretched, in many cases, beyond its capacity to cope. The result is that many children are crying out for attention. They are overweight and under-nourished, lacking in communication skills, and look to TV as their teacher and source of inspiration. Because we are all looking for the answers to living a better life and we want the best for our children, we may ask, "Where do we go from here? What are the answers to help our children?"

Giving our children time, love and tenderness is the best kind of care and attention. You'll be surprised how these three can turn your children around in short time.

Devoting precious time to your children is paramount. Start by turning off the TV. Then sit down with your children and just talk. In our house, I moved the furniture so that the TV is isolated from the main gathering area of the family room. How refreshing and wonderful it is to talk, read, and be together without the intrusive TV. Declare a family night with no TV and eat together and just "be" with your kids. We all want attention, and that is one way to give it to your children and to each other.

The violence on TV has been directly linked to increased violent behavior at school. Our kids are taught by TV that the way to solve a problem is to punch somebody. This shows up later on the playground at school and in the classroom. It seems to be the norm these days to hear about guns, knives, and drugs in every school district in America.

Another TV menace is comedy shows which purport to be the best example of family life and how to communicate in the family unit. Children witness players with clever demeaning dialogue designed to undermine other family members, and it is called healthy and wholesome. Nothing could be further from the truth. Don't get me wrong. I love a good comedy show once in a while (*I Love Lucy* was the best). But I detest programs that belittle, degrade, and make small the tested virtues that have built character over the years. Name me a comedy program that does that today. Instead, we get smart remarks that deprecate sincere, everlasting values, and who is affected? The kids, of

~ ~

course, who are not mature enough to make good judgments for themselves.

Love

Everything I recommended in the nutrition section of this book is true for kids, too! Why am I putting nutrition under love? Because it takes true "tough love" sometimes to stay strong on good nutrition for your children. Also, I don't know any better way to show your kids you love them in the end than by making sure they grow up nutritionally strong and sound from the beginning.

Get your children off junk food. Your child may be full, but is she/he nourished? Children today are typically undernourished. If you don't buy it, they can't eat it! Yes, I know they beg for what they've seen on TV, but when you start feeding your children some of the herbs and nutritional foods I have written about, their cravings for the junk will stop and you will truly find that they don't want it anymore. It is true! Their taste buds, just like yours, will change. Remember, herbs are food, and kids can eat herbs just like you and I. I strongly suggest a good herbal/vitamin/mineral/antioxidant supplemental program for children. And that includes more than just a cartoon-type once-a-day vitamin. There are several herbal companies that have wonderful herbal programs just for children.

One of the reasons we humans, big and small, have cravings is that when we eat the junk, our bodies have not been nourished, and they keep sending signals to eat because they hope we will put something of value in them. In other words, we are craving nourishment. Most of the packaged lunches in the store are convenient but are high in fat and low in nutrition. Did you know that many manufacturers put more fat in the children's food they make than they do in food for adults? And the adults' food has enough fat already. I'm told that one well-known manufacturer that sells pre-made french toast puts 10 percent fat in the adult variety and 14 percent fat in the kids' french toast. Do the manufacturers really believe that kids will eat more french toast because it has more fat in it? Children are

~ ~

not born craving fat. We all need a certain amount in our diets, but we need the good fats, not the bad ones, that show up in so many of the pre-made, processed foods on the market. Another manufacturer that makes a pre-made lunch package for kids puts twenty-eight percent grams of fat in the product. Because there is so much fat and so little nourishment in many of these so-called foods, obesity in children has doubled in the last twenty-five years in this country. Another alarming statistic is that in the U.S. twenty-seven million children under the age of nineteen have high cholesterol levels. Science has found that by the age of ten, children in this country already have arteries and blood vessels which have started to fill with plaque.

Another culprit is sugar. It causes all kinds of problems in children and adults such as cavities, behavioral disorders, and obesity. Limit the foods high in sugar in your house. You may think because you don't allow your children to eat much candy that you are keeping them protected from the effects of too much sugar. However, did you know that 96 percent of calories in cranberry sauce come from sugar? One twelve-ounce regular soda contains approximately ten teaspoons of sugar, one piece of cake contains approxi-

~ ~

mately six teaspoons of sugar, one candy bar contains four teaspoons of sugar, and 63 percent of catsup's calories are from sugar. When you remove white sugar and artificial sweeteners from the diet of a child, you will see a shift in his/her disposition in about three days. The safe sweeteners, and the only ones I recommend, are maple syrup or pure raw honey. I have read dozens of testimonials from parents who have made the switch by removing sugars and products high in sugar in their house, and it works. Also, it is a good idea to eliminate products from your home which have artificial color in them, such as in some fruit punches, sodas, and cereals.

Another important food area that deserves your attention is dairy products. If your child has frequent colds, sore throats, allergy attacks and respiratory problems, you may want to dramatically reduce the dairy and white sugars from his diet. There are good substitutes such as soy milk, almond milk and rice milk that taste great and are nutritionally sound.

If you provide sound, good nutrition for your children, you will soon see positive changes in their health and behavior. Put the herbs to work in your children's bodies, and you will hardly believe the wonderful difference. You will see clarity, concentration

~ ~

and improved communication from your child. It takes time to have a child, and it takes time to love and nourish a child the right way.

Tenderness

There is much to be said for extra tenderness these days, especially in raising children, since kids are often confused by conflicting ideas that come from the media. They need parents who are firm, loving and authoritative, but tender with discipline. I've made a list of things you may wish to do for your kids:

- Invest in quality time with your children every day.
- Offer unconditional love.
- Listen to your children. Really listen.
- Be consistent and fair with discipline with your children.
- Help your children develop and understand the coping skills of life: talking, listening, focusing, organizing, working, socializing, handling stress, playing, and relaxing.
- Teach your children how to love.
- Let your children be children.
- Teach your children responsibility for themselves.

~ ~

- Maintain high expectations for your children.
- Forgive your children instantly when they make mistakes.
- Set the example of how to live, every day, with your children.
- Keep your commitments with your children.
- Walk your talk in everything you do with your children.
- Remember children are a gift from God. Your children are your greatest teachers.

ADD/ADHD — A Sign of Our Times?

I have a personal interest in two childhood diseases which seem to be on the rise. They are Attention Deficit Disorder (ADD) and Attention Deficit Hyperactivity Disorder (ADHD). Today three-and-a-half million children have been diagnosed with ADD. Twice as many boys are diagnosed with ADD/ADHD than girls. Thirty-five percent of the children have siblings with the trait, and 50 percent of ADD children become ADD adults. Too many times when a child needs extra attention, is overactive, easily distracted, or seems to have a behavior problem, he may carry a note

~ ~

from school advising his parents to put their child on a drug called Ritalin. Statistics report that in some schoolrooms across America as many as 50 percent of the children are taking Ritalin. Parents are at a loss as to what to do. Many times children are not adequately tested before a prescription is given out. No one seems to know what causes ADD/ADHD. There are many theories about the root cause, including diet, chemicals or genetics. It is very interesting to me that the symptoms of ADD/ADHD match almost point for point the symptoms of malnutrition. Science has yet to discover the true answer. The result is that some children who are diagnosed ADD or ADHD do not have the disease, and other children who are diagnosed ADD or ADHD have other behavioral challenges instead. Now there is no question that some ADD/ADHD children's symptoms are helped by the drug. But remember, it is a drug, and no one seems to know the long-term effects this drug will have on our children as they grow older. Ritalin is also in the same classification of drugs as cocaine.

As a member of the advisory board of Parents Against Ritalin, it should be quite obvious that I am against the drug. This is because I have become

~ ~

convinced there is still much to be learned about Ritalin, and until the answers are in, I believe herbs may serve as a healthy substitute.

My philosophy about any unproved or questionable drug is not to use it if there is the potential for harm to the user. You may ask, why should Ritalin be the subject of a section in my book, and I must answer it is because I became convinced of the danger of the drug by Debra and Doug Jones. They are the couple who founded PAR, Parents Against Ritalin, because they were concerned about the side effects of the drug.

I've been told that the short-term side effects include loss of appetite, insomnia, decreased growth, anorexia, tachycardia, hypersensitivity, palpitations, nausea, depkinesia, angina, arrhythmia, social withdrawal, abdominal pain, increased heart rate, visual disturbances, psychotic-like symptoms, nervousness, depression, tics, and irritability. No one knows fully what side effects may develop in the future. This information comes from the *Journal of Child and Adolescent Psychopharmacology*. The drug insert that accompanies the medication states that it is not to be given unless environmental causes of the problem have been ruled out. You may have to request this insert from your pharmacist.

~ ~

There are many challenges our children face in today's world — ADD/ADHD is one of them. No matter what the challenge may be, I believe there are answers in these words: **"Time, Love, and Tenderness."**

9

Ingredients for Life

~ ~ ~ ~ ~ ~ ~ ~ ~ ~ ~ ~ ~ ~

*Not knowing when the dawn will come I
open every door.*
— *Emily Dickinson*

*The flowers of all our tomorrows are in the
seeds of today.*
— *Chinese Proverb*

Creating the life you desire is similar to making a culinary masterpiece in your kitchen. The better the ingredients, the better the creation. When you bake a special dish in the kitchen, there is a very special

~ ~

process you follow to make sure it turns out just the way you want. While you are baking, the kitchen may get messy. It may resemble chaos, yet there is order in the process. Life is like that, too. Below are some simple ideas for you to use as ingredients in the creation of your dreams.

Use Fresh, Naturally Grown Nutrients

- You are perfect, just the way you are.
- You were born that way.
- Believe in who you really are.
- Stay fresh and alive by taking better care of you.
- Feed your body, mind, and spirit the nutrients they need every day.
- Treat your body as a temple.

Mix Well and Blend

- Keep balance in your life.
- Play.
- Develop your talents.
- Follow your heart.
- Feel your emotions.
- Laugh a lot.

~ ~

- Cry when you need to.
- Tell the truth.
- Take time for you.
- Be happy. It is a state of mind.
- Surround yourself with people you love and enjoy.

Let Rise

- Stay centered.
- Sleep when you need it.
- Read.
- Write.
- Pray.
- Grow.
- Dream.
- Meditate.
- Be thankful.
- Relax.
- Just be.

Serve Warm

- Be joyful.
- Live in the moment.
- Stay fresh.

~ ~

- Take action when your intuition tells you.
- Let your spirit be your guide; it is your connection to the Divine.
- Keep the love alive inside.

Share With the Community Called Mankind

- No one is an island.
- Be at peace.
- Give your fellow human being a hand.
- Find a cause and give of yourself.
- Be who you really are.
- Accept others the way they are.
- Lead by example.
- Never hold back.
- Forgive everyone, including yourself.
- Make new friends and take good care of the old ones.
- Love your neighbor as yourself.
- Love yourself first or you'll have no love to give away.
- Live your dreams.

଼ ଼ ଼

~ ~

Namasté

I honor the place in you in which the entire Universe dwells. I honor the place in you of love, of light, of truth, and of peace. When you are in that place in you and I am in that place in me, together we are one.

— Universal peace prayer

೮ ೮ ೮

I wish you joy, and I wish you a long, healthy, and happy life, but most of all I wish you love. Go in peace and walk in the light of love.

— Barb Schwarz

~ ~

Epilogue

~ ~ ~ ~ ~ ~ ~ ~ ~ ~ ~ ~ ~ ~

This is Not the End ...
It is Just the Beginning ...

This epilogue is to lift you up. It is here for you to read and reread for your own pure joy. These are thoughts, saying, and poems that I have loved for years. Carry this little book in your briefcase or purse as an inspiration and refer to this section when you are stuck in traffic or taking a break at work, or whenever you need a lift.

Enjoy!

~ ~

Vision is the art of seeing things invisible.
– *Jonathan Swift*

৪ ৪ ৪

Until one is committed, there is hesitancy, the chance to draw back, always ineffectiveness. Concerning all acts of initiative (and creation), there is one elementary truth the ignorance of which kills countless ideas and splendid plans: the moment one definitely commits oneself, then providence moves too.

All sorts of things occur to help one that would never otherwise have occurred. A whole stream of events issues from the decision, raising in one's favor all manner of unforeseen incidents and meetings and material assistance, which no man could have dreamed would have come his way.

– *Goethe*

৪ ৪ ৪

Whatever you can do, or dream you can, begin it. Boldness has genius, power, and magic in it. Begin it now.
– *Goethe*

~ ~

ℬ ℬ ℬ

There are four people named Everybody, Somebody,
Anybody, and Nobody.
There was an important job to be done
And Everybody was asked to do it.
Everybody was sure Somebody would do it.
Anybody could have done it, but Nobody did it.
Somebody got angry about that because it was
Everybody's job.
Everybody thought that Anybody could do it.
But Nobody realized that Everybody would not do it.
It ended up that Everybody blamed Somebody
When Nobody did what Anybody could have done.
– Unknown

ℬ ℬ ℬ

It cannot be when the root is neglected that
what should spring from it will be well ordered.
– Confucius

ℬ ℬ ℬ

~ ~

Community

Next spring when you see geese heading north for the summer, flying along in a "V" formation, you might ponder on how they fly the way they do. It has been learned that as each bird flaps its wings, it creates an uplift for the bird immediately following. By flying in a "V" formation, the whole flock adds at least 71 percent greater flying range than if each goose flew on its own. Whenever a goose falls out of formation, it suddenly feels the drag and resistance of trying to go it alone, and quickly falls back into formation to take advantage of the lifting power of the goose immediately in front.

(People who share a common direction and sense of community can get where they are going quicker and easier, because they are traveling on the thrust of one another.)

When a goose gets sick, two geese fall out of formation and follow him down to help and protect him. They stay with him until he is well again and able to fly. Then they launch out together in formation to catch up with their flock. When the lead goose gets tired he rotates back in the wing and another goose flies point.

~ ~

The geese honk from behind to encourage each other to keep up their effort and speed.

(Through teamwork and words of encouragement given to each other, together we gain strength, courage, and direction.)

– Unknown

(paraphrased by Barb Schwarz)

⅋ ⅋ ⅋

Success

Start with a dream (vision)
Unlock any negative thinking
Courage of your convictions (goals)
Commitment (be accountable)
Enthusiasm (practice it)
Spiritualize (let go ... let God)
Stick with it (never give up)

– Unknown

⅋ ⅋ ⅋

If you do not change your beliefs in your life, your life will be like it is forever.

– Barb Schwarz

~ ~

℘ ℘ ℘

Because I am the only person I will have a relationship with all of my life, I choose:
- To love myself the way I am now
- To always acknowledge that I am enough just the way I am
- To love, honor and cherish myself
- To be my own best friend
- To be the person I would like to spend the rest of my life with
- To always take care of myself so that I can take care of others
- To always grow, develop and share my love and life.

– *Ron and Mary Hulnick*

℘ ℘ ℘

Best vitamin for making friends: B1
– *Unknown*

℘ ℘ ℘

~ ~

Awakening

Spring's voice may still be a whisper
as winter wanes,
but the earth is pulsating with life!
Ground that has long looked bare
will soon send forth new life!

Like the earth,
I awaken to the unlimited possibilities
that life holds.
I explore new ideas,
experience new feelings,
and embrace the wonder of discovery
that is stirring within me
and around me.

I weed out old ideas and feelings
that prevent me from enjoying
the entire landscape of possibilities.
I clear the way for the growth
of new ideas and feelings,
I nurture them so that
they take root and thrive.

~ ~

Spring is a season of the Earth,
but more importantly,
it is a time of awakening to
new and wonder-filled possibilities.

I awaken to the spring of my soul.
– Unknown

୫ ୫ ୫

*What you make of what you have been
given is who you become.*
– Unknown

୫ ୫ ୫

Blessings

Believe and expect to receive.
In your asking trust.
As you trust be thankful.
Thanksgiving brings abundance.
Now, let go and know
that spirit is working through you.
And that, is the greatest blessing of all.
– Barb Schwarz

~ ~

 ⅋ ⅋ ⅋

Love
Love is patient and kind.
It doesn't envy or boast
and it's never proud.

It's not rude or selfish,
it doesn't get angry easily
or keep track of wrong.

Love doesn't delight in bad things,
but it rejoices in the truth.
Love always protects,
trusts, hopes, and perseveres.

Love never fails.
– 1 Corinthians 13

 ⅋ ⅋ ⅋

A laugh is an instant vacation.
– Unknown

 ⅋ ⅋ ⅋

~ ~

Take God as Your Partner

Why not organize the business of living in a big way?

Why creep along, as some people do, from one tiny stepping-stone to another, instead of striding out boldly? Why be content with poor health, uninteresting work, or restricted conditions, when many other people have already risen above these things?

There is a way out of limitation that never fails. It is simple. It calls for no formalities. It requires no money. It is obvious enough when you realize it; but it is strange how many people nevertheless overlook it. It is this, take God for your partner.

If you will really make God your business partner in every department of your life, you will be amazed at the quick and striking results that you will obtain.

Of course, if you want God to be your partner, He/She will have to be the Senior Partner, and you will have to include Him/Her in every corner and every phase of your life. If you are prepared to do this, the result will not be in doubt.

Most people would be thrilled to be able to go into partnership with some great industrial or financial

~ ~

magnate: they would feel that their future was assured. But here is a partnership with Infinite Power awaiting you. Take God as Your Partner.

– Ralph Waldo Emerson

଼ ଼ ଼

Kabir says, "Student tell me, what is God?"
The student replies, "God is the breath inside the breath."

– Kabir

଼ ଼ ଼

Breathe in spirit ... breathe out love ... breathe in spirit ... breathe out love.

– Barb Schwarz

଼ ଼ ଼

What you give keeps, what you keep spoils.

– Unknown

଼ ଼ ଼

~ ~

⅋ ⅋ ⅋

Forgiveness Program
Sunday forgive yourself
Monday forgive your family
Tuesday forgive your friends
Wednesday forgive your business associates
Thursday forgive across economic lines
Friday forgive across political lines
Saturday forgive across cultural lines.

– Barb Schwarz

⅋ ⅋ ⅋

*To know and not to do ... is not really yet
to know.*

– Chinese Proverb

⅋ ⅋ ⅋

*Don't be pushed by your problems, be led
by your dreams.*

– Unknown

~ ~

❦ ❦ ❦

From: A Return to Love

Our deepest fear is not that we are inadequate.
Our deepest fear is that we are powerful beyond
measure.
It is our light, not our darkness, that most frightens us.
We ask ourselves, Who am I to be brilliant, gorgeous,
talented, fabulous?
Actually, who are you not to be?
You are a child of God.
Your playing small doesn't serve the world.
There's nothing enlightened about shrinking so that
other people won't feel insecure around you.
We are all meant to shine, as children do.
We were born to make manifest the glory of God that
is within us.
It is not just in some of us; it is in everyone.
And as we let our own light shine, we unconsciously
give other people permission to do the same.
As we are liberated from our own fear, our presence
automatically liberates others.

– Marianne Williamson

~ ~

The true joy of life is being used for a purpose recognized by yourself as a mighty one.

— George Bernard Shaw

ଙ ଙ ଙ

Care more than others think is wise,
Risk more than other think is safe,
Expect more than others think is possible and
Dream more than others think is practical.

— Barb Schwarz

ଙ ଙ ଙ

Today

I am younger today than I was yesterday.
I am wiser in spirit and mind.
My body is healed and in a perfect state of health.
There is no fear in my mind and there is love in my life
and all around me.
The Universe's eternal river of energy and abundance is
flowing to me.
I am a crucial part of the collective consciousness of
this universe, because I am a child of God.

— Barb Schwarz

The Illustrators

~ ~ ~ ~ ~ ~ ~ ~ ~ ~ ~ ~ ~ ~

Andrea Schwarz

Andrea Schwarz is my daughter. She is one of the most beautiful people I have ever met. This is not just because she is my daughter, but rather because of the person she is and the joy she brings to all around her. When Andrea was eighteen years old she was a model, an A student, and a downhill skier. Because of an automobile accident in which she was the passenger, she became brain damaged and mentally ill. She has worked with her illness and mental challenges for the last six years, and she has made miraculous growth in her healing. Three years ago it was very difficult for her to

~ ~

put a piece of paper into an envelope, even though she would try for hours. Today she works in our warehouse for three days a week, and it is hard to get her to take a break.

I am honored to have my daughter do the sketches for this book. When her art therapy began five-and-a-half years ago, she drew scribbles and X's on the papers like a preschooler would do. Now you see her progress and her lovely work in this book. Miracles do happen.

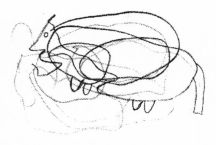

This is one of the pictures that Andrea drew a year after her accident in her class with her art therapist Margaret Carpenter. You can tell how far Andrea has come as you see the pictures she drew for this book.

Andrea is one of the main reasons for my passion for the herbs. The herbal program we have used for her has touched her life and ours in a way that words cannot describe. She continues on her path to wellness, and there is great truth in the statement that there can be miraculous healings through herbs. This book has

~ ~

evolved as a part of my growth, as well as hers because Andrea is my greatest teacher. I am blessed to have her as my daughter. I hope you enjoy her beautiful drawings.

Margaret Carpenter

Margaret Carpenter came into our lives like an angel. She has worked with Andrea as her art therapist for over five years, since Andrea's accident. She is patient, kind, loving, and talented. Her soft English accent puts anyone at ease immediately. Margaret is a graduate nurse, an art therapist and a professional artist. She has a private practice in Seattle, Washington, and she continues to show and sell her paintings in galleries in California and Washington. Her work is currently represented at The Kirsten Gallery in Seattle.

In this book Margaret worked with Andrea in the development of Andrea's drawings. She continues to touch my daughter's life, and mine as well, in very special gifted ways. Margaret also drew the inspiring symbol for the body, mind, and spirit chapters. Thank you Margaret for your love and care.

Barb Schwarz, CSP, is a renowned international speaker. She is known for her ability to educate, enlighten, and entertain. To bring Barb to your company or organization, call her office.

Barb's Life-Changing Tools

Barb's audio and video programs change people's lives. For a complete list of her latest work, please call her office.

Barb's Herbal Nutritional Program

To order Barb Schwarz's recommended herbal nutritional program for weight loss and/or to bring your body into nutritional balance, call her office.

Newsletter

For a free copy of Barb's herbal health newsletter call her office.

Barb's office:
206-391-2272 or 1-800-392-7161

To order additional copies of

If You Wear Out Your Body, Where Will You Live?

Book: $12.95   Shipping/Handling $3.00

Contact:

BookPartners, Inc.

P.O. Box 922
Wilsonville, Oregon 97070

Fax: 503-682-8684
Phone: 1-800-895-7323